Book Title: "Is Expensive Coffee Actually Worth It?"

By Jenny Koo

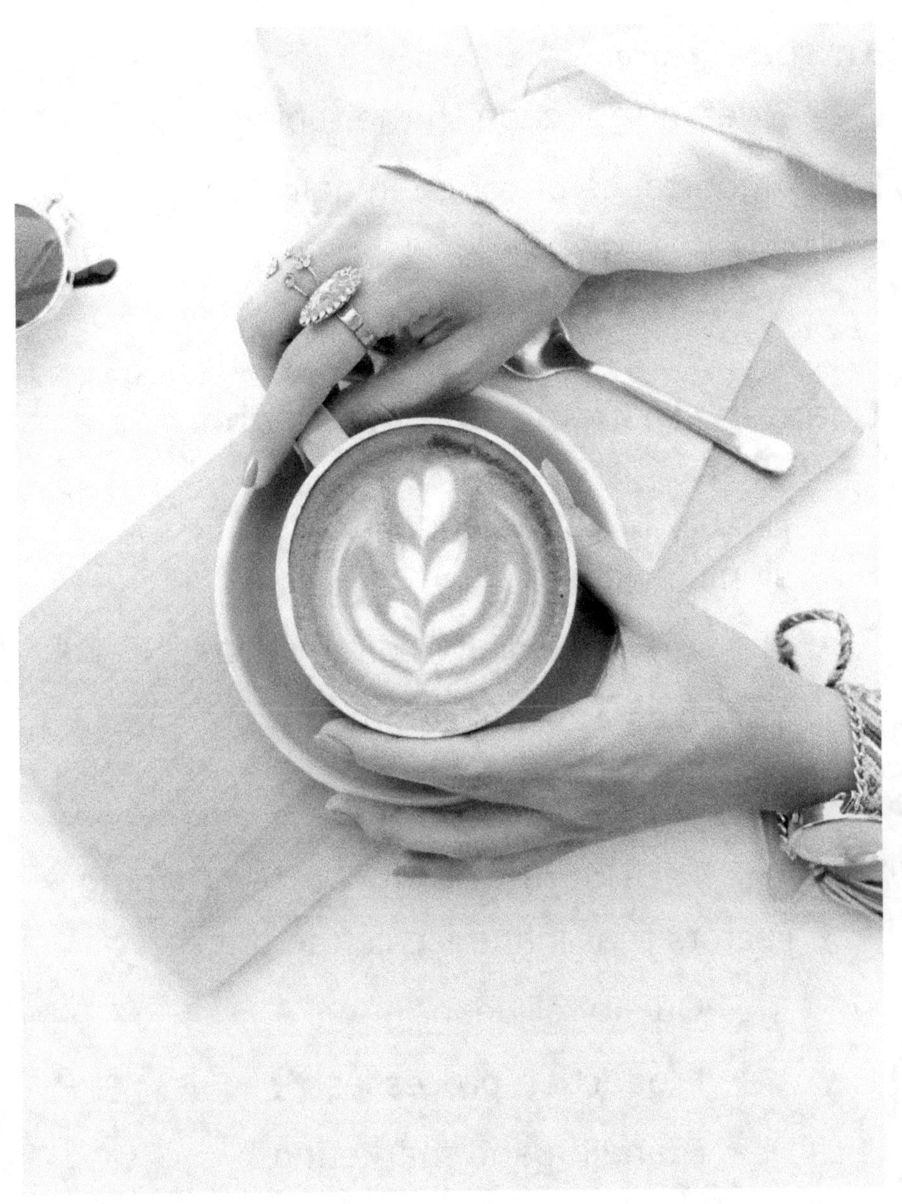

Introduction

- Brief introduction to the topic
- Importance of coffee in daily life
- Purpose of this book

Chapter 1: The Coffee Culture and Economy

- History of coffee and its cultural significance
- The rise of specialty coffee shops
- Coffee as a global commodity

Chapter 2: Understanding Coffee Pricing

- Factors that influence coffee prices
    - Quality of beans
    - Production processes
    - Branding and marketing
- Comparing expensive and inexpensive coffee brands

Chapter 3: The Science Behind Coffee Quality

- Types of coffee beans: Arabica vs. Robusta

- The impact of growing conditions and regions

- Processing methods: Washed vs. natural

Chapter 4: Brewing Methods and Their Impact on Cost

- Popular brewing methods (e.g., espresso, pour-over, French press)

- Equipment and tools: Basic vs. high-end

- How brewing methods affect flavor and price

Chapter 5: The Role of Baristas and Cafés

- Skills and expertise of baristas

- The ambiance and experience of high-end cafés

- Case studies of renowned coffee shops

Chapter 6: Health Benefits and Risks of Coffee Consumption

- Nutritional content of coffee

- Benefits of moderate coffee consumption

- Potential risks and downsides

Chapter 7: Consumer Perception and Psychology

- The psychology of luxury and status symbols

- Why people choose expensive coffee

- The influence of marketing and social media

Chapter 8: Is Expensive Coffee Environmentally Sustainable?

- Sustainability practices in the coffee industry

- Certifications: Fair Trade, Organic, Rainforest Alliance

- The environmental impact of high-end vs. mass-produced coffee

Chapter 9: Personal Preferences and Taste Tests

- Conducting blind taste tests
- Analyzing taste preferences across price ranges
- Stories and testimonials from coffee enthusiasts

Conclusion

- Summary of findings
- Final thoughts on the value of expensive coffee
- Encouragement for readers to explore and decide for themselves

References

- Comprehensive list of sources and further reading

Recommended Reading List

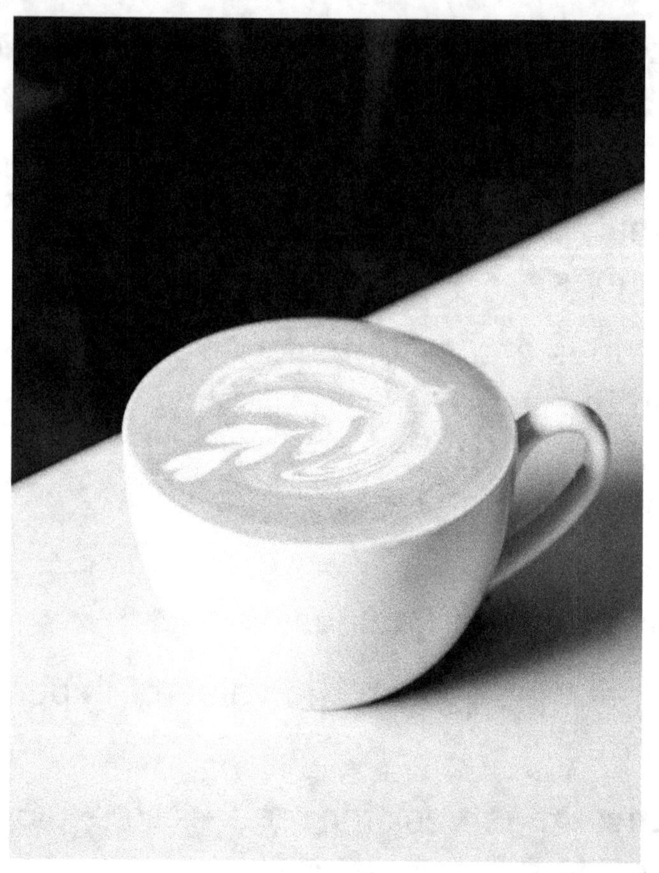

Introduction

Coffee is more than just a beverage; it's a global phenomenon with deep-rooted cultural significance and a thriving economy. Whether it's a morning ritual, a social lubricant, or a subject of gourmet discussion, coffee holds a unique place in our lives. But as the coffee industry has evolved, so too have the prices of our favorite caffeinated drinks. This ebook delves into the intriguing question: Is expensive coffee actually worth it?

We will explore the various facets of the coffee world, from the history and culture of coffee drinking to the intricate science behind coffee quality and brewing methods. We'll examine the factors that contribute to the cost of coffee, including the skills of baristas and the experience offered by high-end cafés. Additionally, we'll look into the health implications of coffee consumption, the psychology behind our buying decisions, and the environmental sustainability of coffee production.

Our journey will be comprehensive, providing insights into whether the price tag on a premium cup of coffee is justified. By the end of this ebook, you'll have a well-rounded understanding of what goes into your cup and be better equipped to decide if that expensive brew is truly worth it.

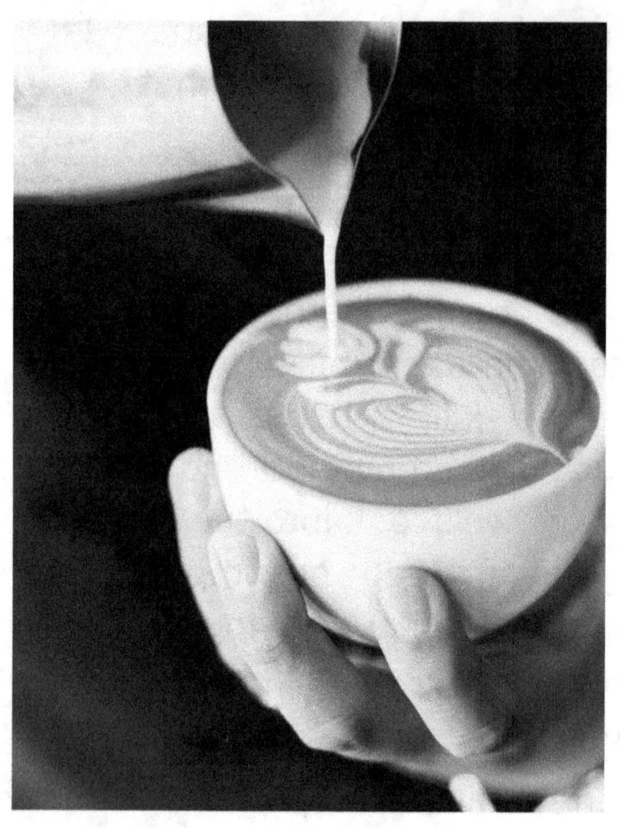

Chapter 1: The Coffee Culture and Economy

History of Coffee and Its Cultural Significance

Coffee's journey from an Ethiopian goat herder's discovery to becoming a staple in modern society is a fascinating one. According to legend, the energizing effects of coffee were first discovered by a shepherd named Kaldi, who noticed his goats became unusually lively after eating the berries of a certain tree. From Ethiopia, coffee spread to the Arabian Peninsula, where it became an integral part of the Islamic world, aiding in long prayer sessions and social gatherings.

In the 16th century, coffee reached Europe, initially met with suspicion but soon becoming the drink of choice in coffee houses that sprang up across the continent. These establishments became hubs for intellectual exchange, earning the nickname "penny universities" for the price of a cup of coffee.

The Rise of Specialty Coffee Shops

The 20th century witnessed the emergence of specialty coffee shops, revolutionizing how we perceive and consume coffee. The first wave of coffee culture focused on making coffee a household staple, with brands like Folgers and Maxwell House leading the charge. The second wave brought us Starbucks and other chains that emphasized consistency and convenience, making espresso drinks mainstream.

The third wave of coffee is characterized by an artisanal approach, emphasizing quality, sourcing, and brewing methods. Specialty coffee shops prioritize transparency and traceability, often sourcing beans directly from farmers and paying premiums for higher quality. This wave has given rise to a coffee culture that values the craftsmanship and experience behind each cup.

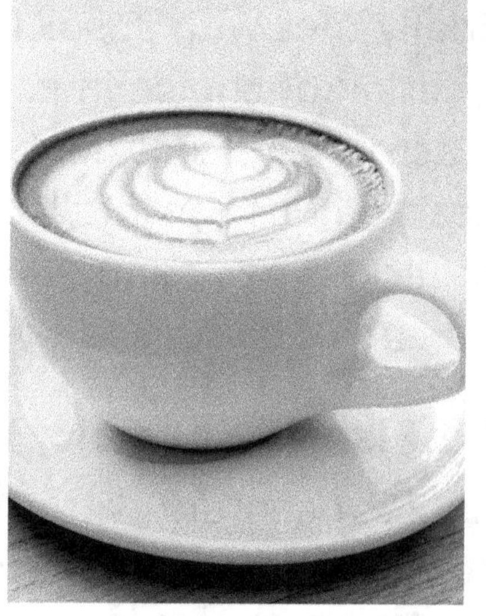

Coffee as a Global Commodity

Coffee is one of the most traded commodities in the world, second only to oil. The global coffee market is worth billions of dollars, with millions of people involved in its cultivation, production, and distribution. Coffee's economic impact is significant, particularly in developing countries where it serves as a primary source of income for many farmers.

Despite its economic importance, the coffee industry faces numerous challenges, including volatile market prices, climate change, and sustainability concerns. These factors contribute to the complexity of coffee pricing and underscore the importance of understanding the value chain from bean to cup.

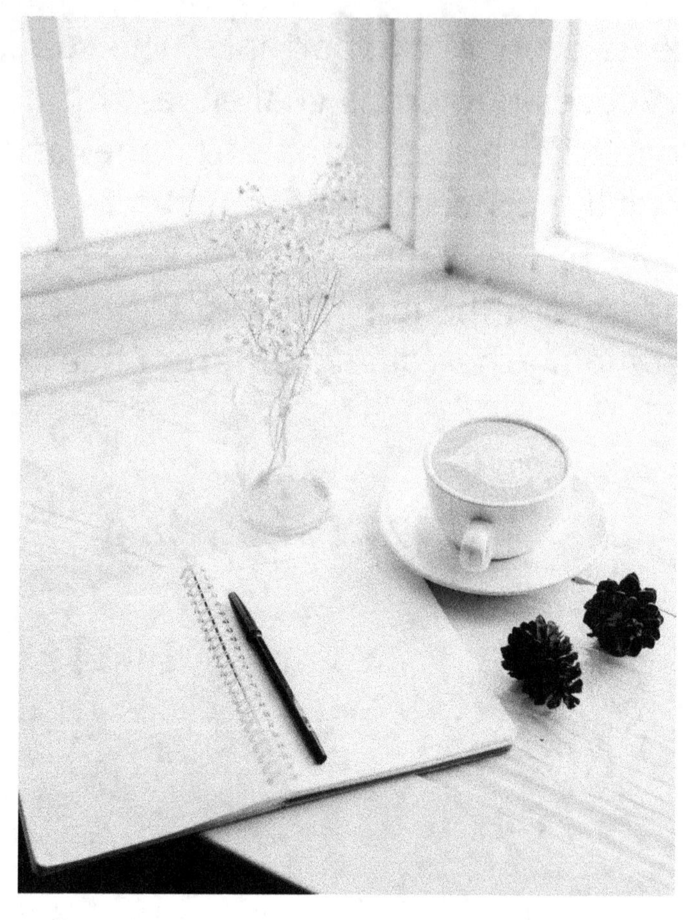

Chapter 2: Understanding Coffee Pricing

Factors That Influence Coffee Prices

The price of coffee can vary widely, influenced by several key factors:

- Quality of Beans: Higher quality beans, typically Arabica, are more expensive due to their superior flavor profiles and more labor-intensive cultivation. Robusta beans, on the other hand, are cheaper but often considered inferior in taste.

- Production Processes: The methods used to process coffee, such as washed or natural processing, can affect the cost. Washed coffees, known for their clarity and brightness, generally command higher prices due to the additional labor and equipment required.

- Branding and Marketing: The perception of a brand can significantly impact the price of coffee. Specialty brands that emphasize sustainability, ethical sourcing, and artisanal craftsmanship often charge a premium.

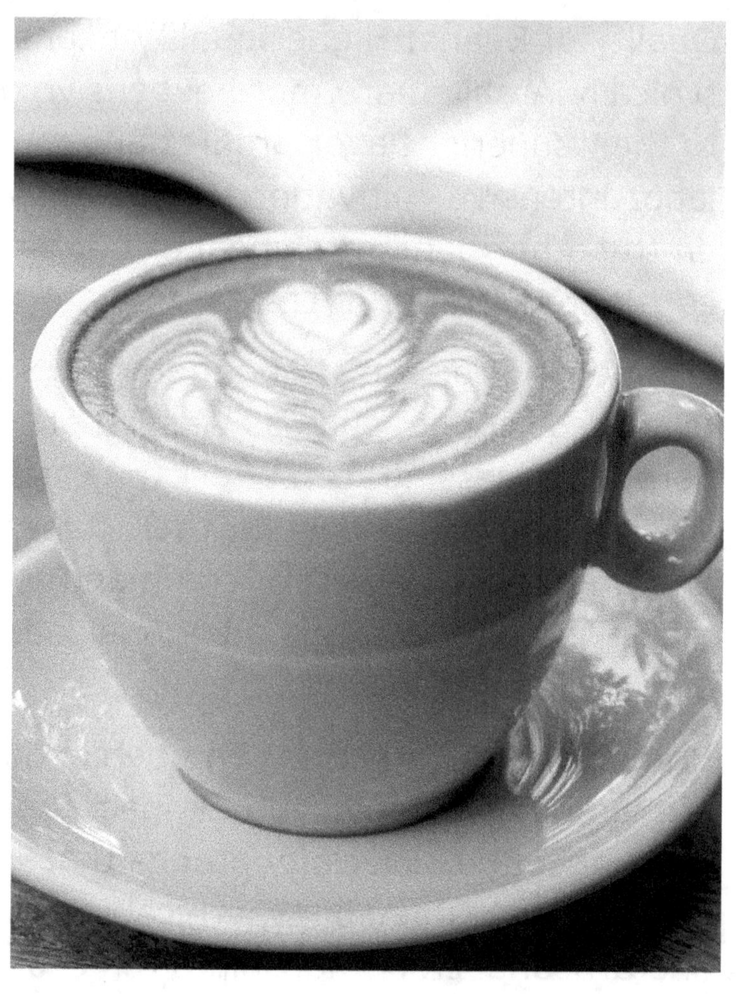

Comparing Expensive and Inexpensive Coffee Brands

When comparing expensive and inexpensive coffee brands, several differences become apparent. High-end brands often invest in better quality control, ensuring consistency in their product. They may also engage in direct trade practices, which involve building relationships with farmers and paying them higher prices for better quality beans.

In contrast, cheaper brands might use lower quality beans and blend them to mask inconsistencies in flavor. They often focus on mass production and cost-cutting measures, which can affect the overall quality of the coffee.

Understanding these differences helps consumers make more informed choices, balancing their budget with their desire for quality and ethical considerations.

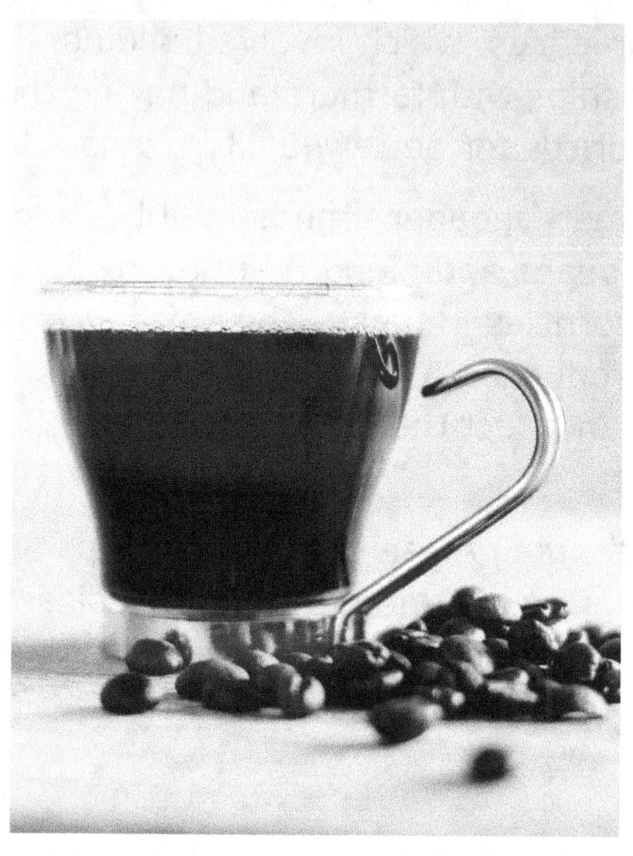

Chapter 3: The Science Behind Coffee Quality

Types of Coffee Beans: Arabica vs. Robusta

Arabica and Robusta are the two primary species of coffee beans, each with distinct characteristics:

- Arabica: Known for its smooth, complex flavors, Arabica beans are grown at higher altitudes and require more care. They have a wider range of taste profiles, including fruity, floral, and nutty notes. Arabica beans are more susceptible to pests and diseases, making them more expensive to cultivate.

- Robusta: These beans are hardier and can be grown at lower altitudes. They have a stronger, more bitter flavor with higher caffeine content. Robusta is often used in blends and instant coffee due to its lower cost and strong flavor profile.

The Impact of Growing Conditions and Regions

The growing conditions and regions where coffee is cultivated play a crucial role in its quality. Factors such as altitude, climate, soil composition, and rainfall influence the flavor profile of the beans. For example, beans grown in high-altitude regions like Ethiopia or Colombia tend to have more acidity and complex flavors, making them highly sought after.

Each coffee-growing region imparts unique characteristics to the beans, known as terroir. This concept, borrowed from the wine industry, highlights the importance of origin in determining the quality and taste of coffee.

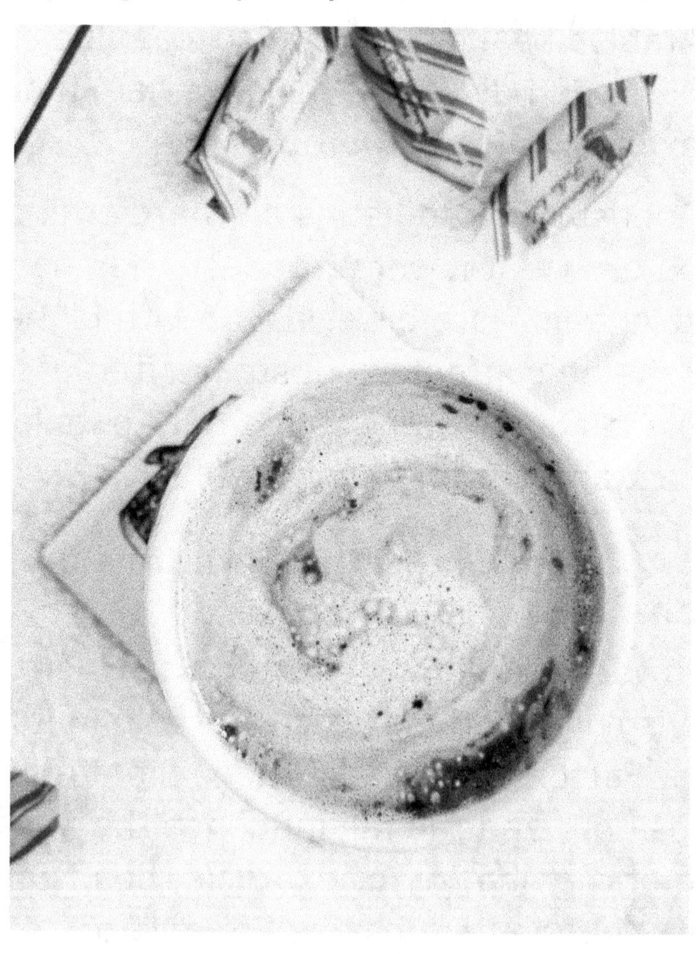

Processing Methods: Washed vs. Natural

Coffee processing methods significantly impact the final flavor of the beans. The two primary methods are:

- Washed (Wet) Processing: This method involves removing the fruit from the beans before drying. It produces cleaner, brighter flavors and is often used for high-quality Arabica beans. The process requires more water and equipment, contributing to higher costs.

- Natural (Dry) Processing: In this method, the beans are dried with the fruit still attached, imparting more fruity and fermented flavors. It requires less water but can result in more inconsistent quality. Natural processing is often used in regions with limited water resources.

Understanding these processing methods helps consumers appreciate the complexity and craftsmanship involved in producing high-quality coffee.

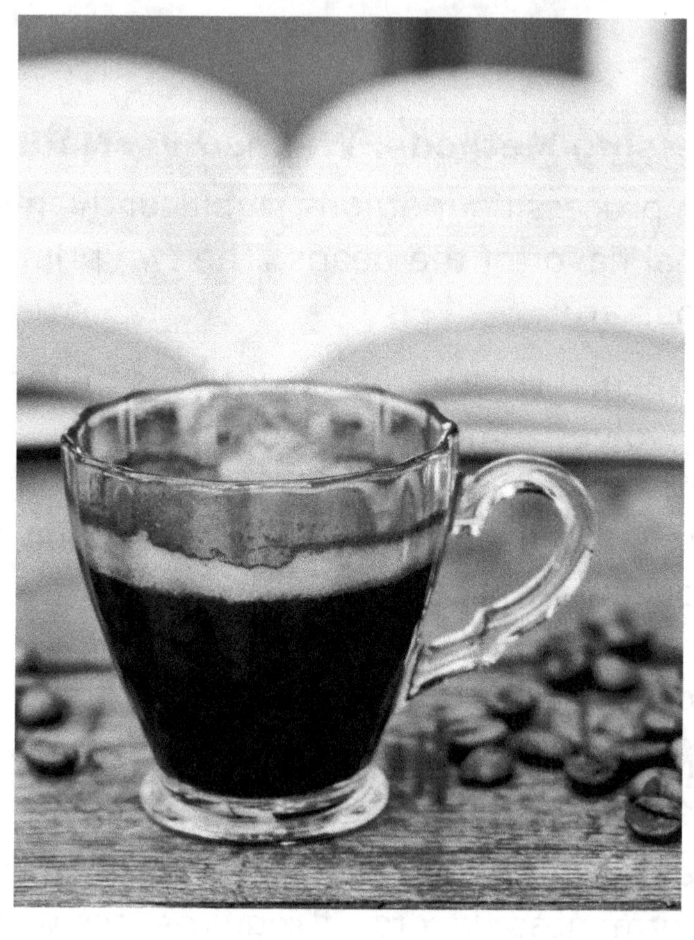

Chapter 4: Brewing Methods and Their Impact on Cost

Popular Brewing Methods

Different brewing methods can significantly affect the flavor and cost of coffee. Some popular methods include:

- Espresso: A concentrated coffee brewed by forcing hot water through finely-ground coffee beans. Espresso machines can be expensive, but they produce rich, flavorful coffee quickly.

- Pour-Over: A manual brewing method that involves pouring hot water over coffee grounds in a filter. It allows for precise control over brewing variables, resulting in a clean and complex cup of coffee.

- French Press: A simple, immersion brewing method that involves steeping coffee grounds in hot water before pressing them with a plunger. It produces a full-bodied and robust cup of coffee.

- Aeropress: A versatile and portable brewing device that uses air pressure to push hot water through coffee grounds. It can produce both espresso-like and regular coffee.

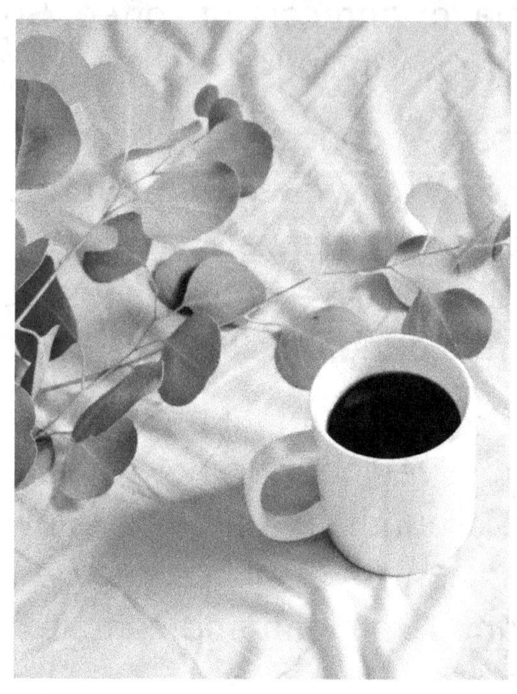

Equipment and Tools: Basic vs. High-End

The cost of brewing coffee can vary depending on the equipment and tools used. Basic equipment, such as a French press or pour-over cone, is relatively inexpensive and can produce excellent coffee. However, high-end equipment like espresso machines, grinders, and precision scales can significantly increase the cost.

Investing in quality equipment can enhance the brewing experience and result in better-tasting coffee. High-end grinders, for example, ensure consistent grind size, which is crucial for optimal extraction and flavor.

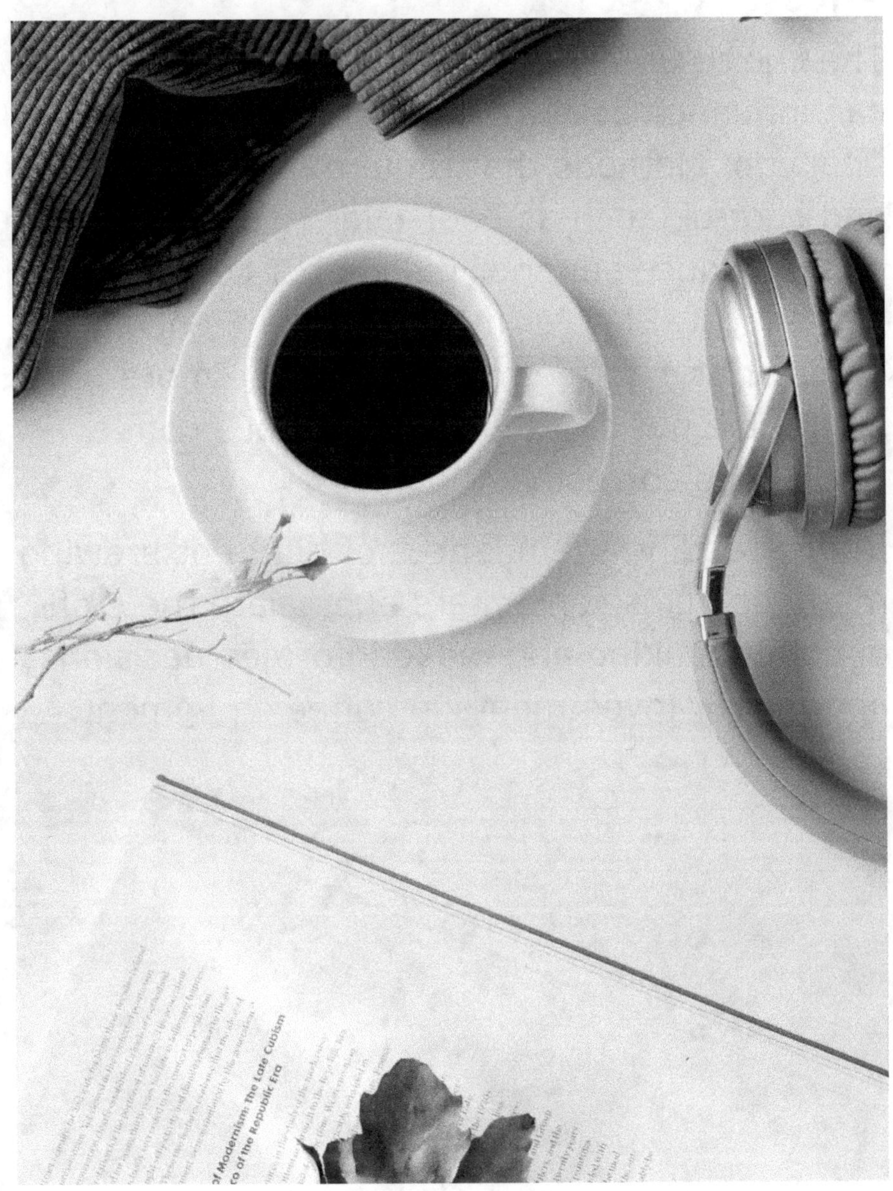

How Brewing Methods Affect Flavor and Price

The choice of brewing method and equipment can influence both the flavor and price of the final cup. Methods that require more precision and control, such as pour-over or espresso, often produce superior results but come at a higher cost. Simpler methods, like French press or drip coffee makers, may be more affordable but can still yield delicious coffee when used correctly.

Understanding the nuances of different brewing methods helps consumers appreciate the craft of coffee making and make informed decisions about their investments in coffee equipment.

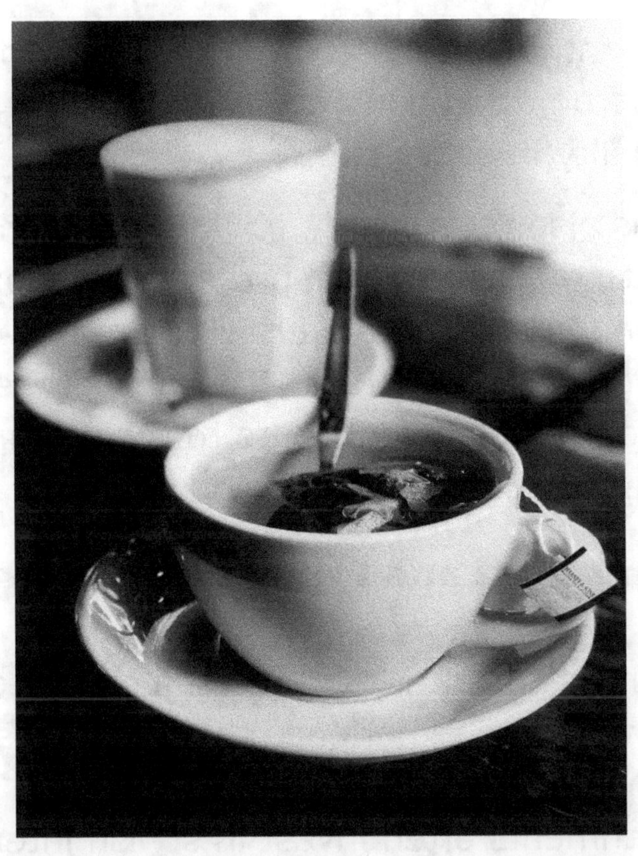

Chapter 5: The Role of Baristas and Cafés

Skills and Expertise of Baristas

Baristas play a crucial role in the coffee experience, bringing expertise and craftsmanship to every cup they prepare. Skilled baristas have a deep understanding of coffee beans, brewing methods, and equipment. They are trained to extract the best flavors from the beans, ensuring consistency and quality in every cup.

Baristas also possess the ability to customize drinks to meet individual preferences, from adjusting grind size and brewing time to creating intricate latte art. Their expertise and attention to detail contribute to the premium experience offered by high-end cafés.

The Ambiance and Experience of High-End Cafés

High-end cafés offer more than just coffee; they provide an experience that combines ambiance, service, and quality. These establishments often invest in stylish interiors, comfortable seating, and a welcoming atmosphere. The attention to detail extends to every aspect of the café, from the choice of music to the presentation of the drinks.

The experience of enjoying a cup of coffee in a high-end café can justify the higher prices. Customers are paying for the ambiance, the expertise of the baristas, and the overall sense of luxury and indulgence.

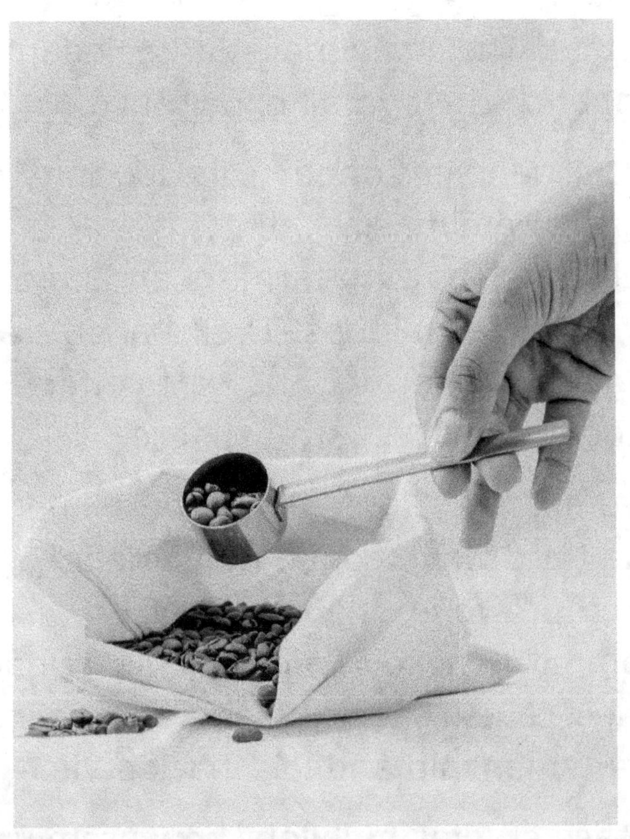

Case Studies of Renowned Coffee Shops

Several renowned coffee shops around the world exemplify the principles of quality and experience. For example:

- Blue Bottle Coffee: Known for its meticulous sourcing and roasting processes, Blue Bottle Coffee has built a reputation for high-quality, freshly roasted coffee. Their minimalist and elegant cafés enhance the overall experience.

- Intelligentsia Coffee: This specialty coffee roaster emphasizes direct trade relationships with farmers and innovative brewing techniques. Their baristas are highly trained, and the cafés offer a modern, inviting atmosphere.

- Stumptown Coffee Roasters: Pioneers of the third wave coffee movement, Stumptown is celebrated for its commitment to quality and sustainability. Their cafés reflect a blend of artisanal craftsmanship and laid-back style.

These case studies highlight how premium coffee shops create value beyond the beverage itself, fostering a culture of appreciation and enjoyment around coffee.

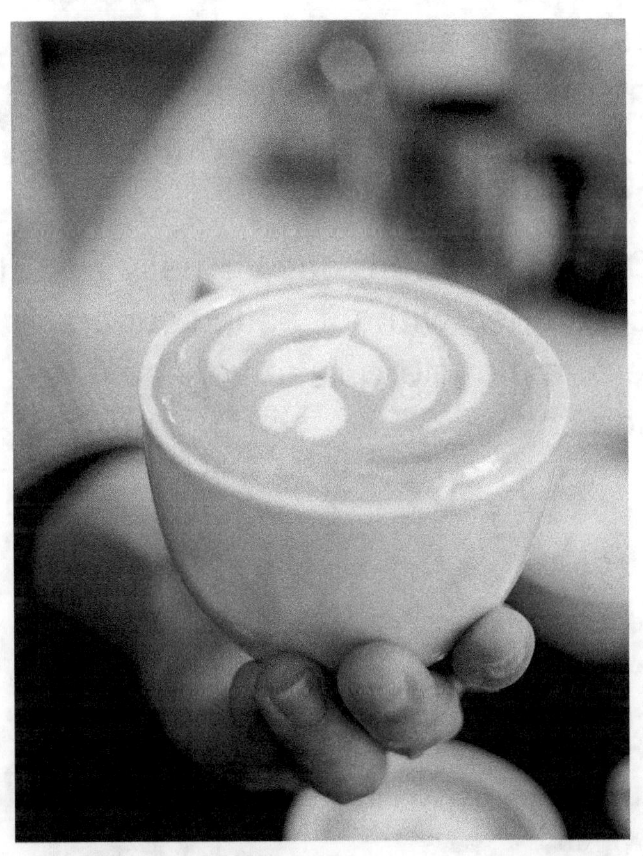

Chapter 6: Health Benefits and Risks of Coffee Consumption

Nutritional Content of Coffee

Coffee is a complex beverage containing numerous compounds that can impact health. It is rich in antioxidants, such as chlorogenic acids, which have been linked to various health benefits. Coffee also contains essential nutrients like vitamins B2 (riboflavin), B3 (niacin), B5 (pantothenic acid), and manganese.

A typical cup of coffee has virtually no calories when consumed without added sugars or creamers, making it a relatively healthy beverage choice.

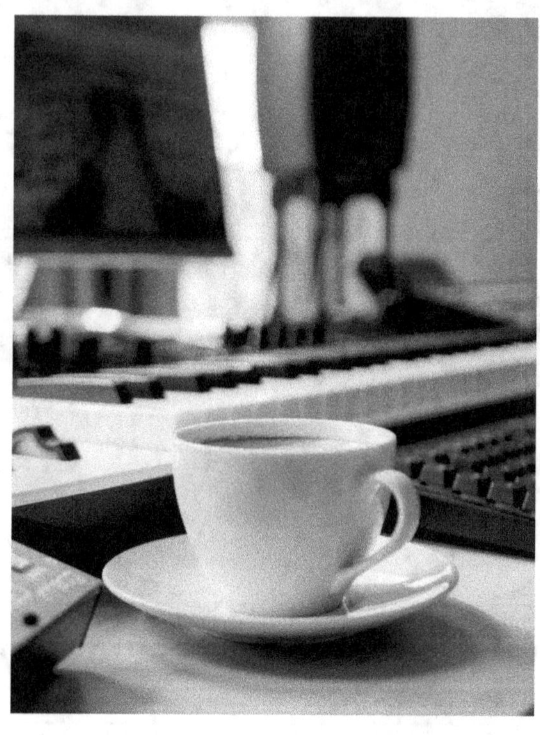

Benefits of Moderate Coffee Consumption

Moderate coffee consumption has been associated with several health benefits, including:

- Improved Cognitive Function: Caffeine, a natural stimulant found in coffee, can enhance alertness, concentration, and overall cognitive function.

- Reduced Risk of Chronic Diseases: Studies suggest that regular coffee consumption may lower the risk of developing conditions such as type 2 diabetes, Parkinson's disease, Alzheimer's disease, and certain types of cancer.

- Cardiovascular Health: Some research indicates that moderate coffee intake can have a protective effect on the heart, reducing the risk of stroke and heart disease.

These benefits are most pronounced with moderate consumption, typically defined as 3-4 cups per day.

Potential Risks and Downsides

While coffee has many health benefits, excessive consumption can lead to adverse effects, including:

- Insomnia and Anxiety: High caffeine intake can disrupt sleep patterns and increase anxiety levels, particularly in sensitive individuals.

- Digestive Issues: Coffee is acidic and can cause stomach discomfort or exacerbate conditions like acid reflux in some people.

- Addiction and Withdrawal: Regular consumption of caffeine can lead to dependence, with withdrawal symptoms such as headaches, fatigue, and irritability when intake is reduced.

Understanding these risks helps consumers make informed decisions about their coffee consumption and maintain a balanced approach to enjoying their favorite beverage.

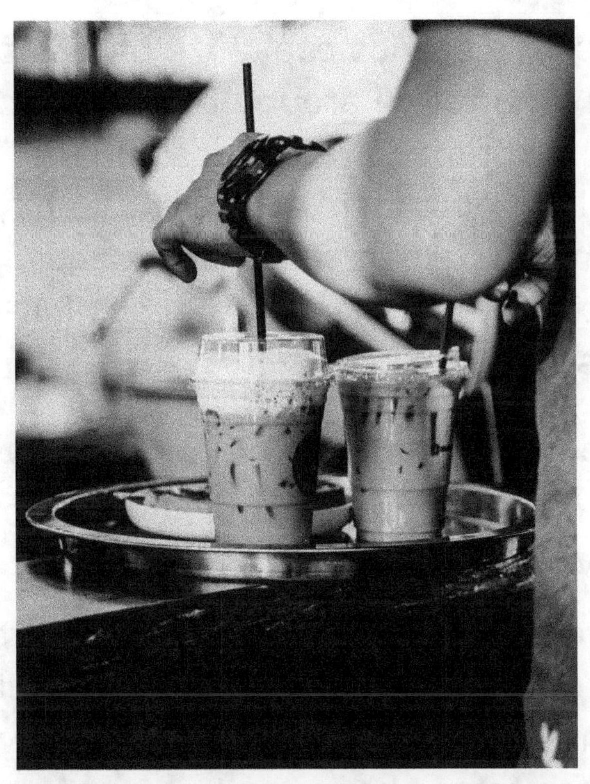

Chapter 7: Consumer Perception and Psychology

The Psychology of Luxury and Status Symbols

Expensive coffee often functions as a status symbol, reflecting a consumer's taste, sophistication, and social standing. The psychology behind luxury goods suggests that people derive pleasure not just from the product itself, but from the perception of exclusivity and the social signals it sends.

Luxury coffee brands capitalize on this by creating a narrative around their products, emphasizing rarity, craftsmanship, and exclusivity. Consumers are willing to pay a premium for the perceived status and satisfaction that comes with these high-end products.

Why People Choose Expensive Coffee

Several factors drive consumers to choose expensive coffee:

- Perceived Quality: Higher prices are often associated with better quality, leading consumers to believe that expensive coffee tastes better or is made from superior beans.

- Ethical Considerations: Many high-end coffee brands emphasize ethical sourcing, sustainability, and fair trade practices. Consumers who prioritize these values are willing to pay more to support responsible production.

- Personal Indulgence: For some, expensive coffee represents a personal treat or indulgence. The ritual of enjoying a well-crafted cup of coffee can be a form of self-care and a way to savor small luxuries in daily life.

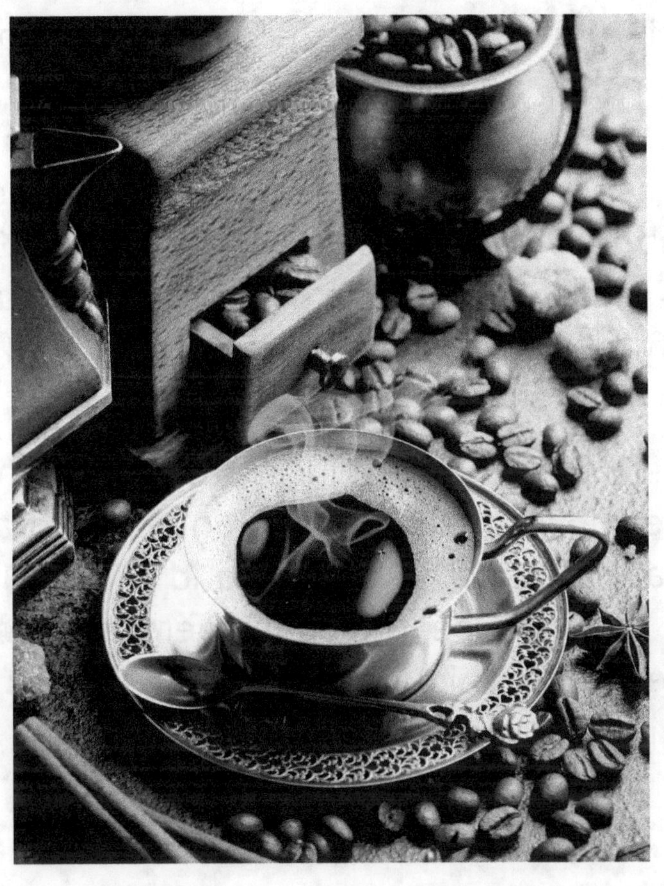

The Influence of Marketing and Social Media

Marketing and social media play significant roles in shaping consumer perceptions of coffee. Influencers and coffee enthusiasts often showcase premium coffee brands, creating aspirational content that drives demand. Social media platforms like Instagram and YouTube amplify the reach of these messages, making luxury coffee more desirable.

Brands also use marketing strategies such as storytelling, limited editions, and collaborations to create a sense of urgency and exclusivity. These tactics appeal to consumers' emotions and desire for unique experiences, further justifying the higher prices.

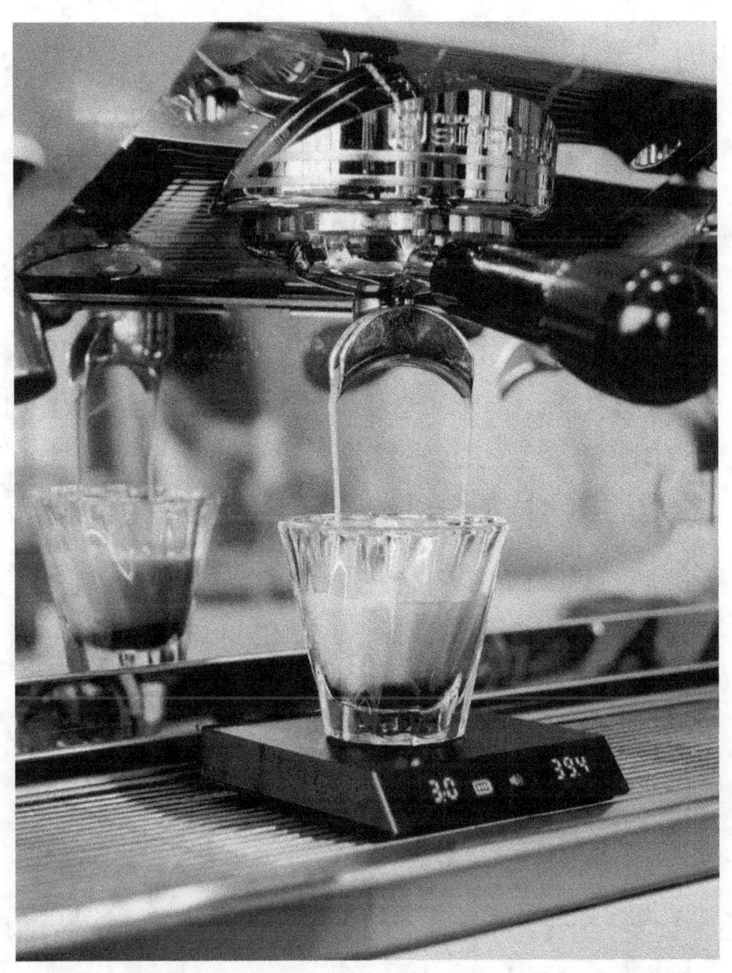

Chapter 8: Is Expensive Coffee Environmentally Sustainable?

Sustainability Practices in the Coffee Industry

Sustainability is a growing concern in the coffee industry, with many high-end brands leading the charge in adopting eco-friendly practices. These practices include:

- Organic Farming: Avoiding synthetic pesticides and fertilizers to protect the environment and improve soil health.

- Shade-Grown Coffee: Cultivating coffee under the canopy of native trees, which promotes biodiversity and reduces the need for deforestation.

- Water Conservation: Implementing methods to reduce water usage during processing, such as using dry or semi-washed techniques.

Certifications: Fair Trade, Organic, Rainforest Alliance

Several certifications help consumers identify sustainably produced coffee, including:

- Fair Trade: Ensures that farmers receive fair prices for their beans, promoting economic stability and ethical labor practices.

- Organic: Certifies that the coffee is grown without synthetic chemicals, supporting environmental health and sustainability.

- Rainforest Alliance: Focuses on conserving biodiversity and promoting sustainable livelihoods for farmers through rigorous environmental and social standards.

These certifications often come with higher costs, reflected in the price of the final product. However, they provide consumers with assurance that their purchase supports sustainable and ethical practices.

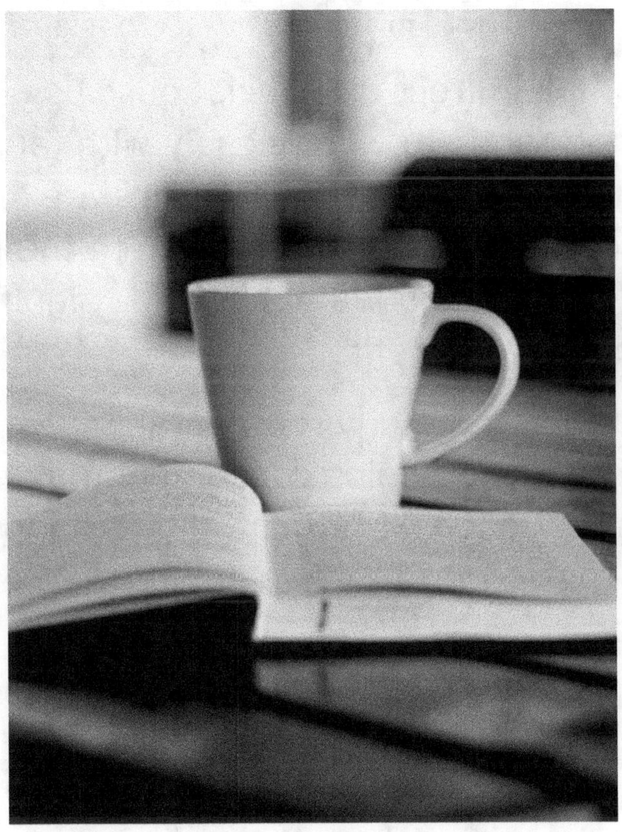

The Environmental Impact of High-End vs. Mass-Produced Coffee

High-end coffee brands tend to emphasize sustainability more than mass-produced counterparts. While mass-produced coffee often focuses on maximizing yield and minimizing costs, leading to practices that can harm the environment, high-end brands invest in sustainable methods that prioritize long-term environmental health.

For example, direct trade relationships allow high-end brands to work closely with farmers, ensuring that sustainable practices are followed. These efforts contribute to the higher cost of premium coffee but provide significant environmental benefits.

Understanding the environmental impact of coffee production helps consumers make choices that align with their values, supporting brands that prioritize sustainability and ethical practices.

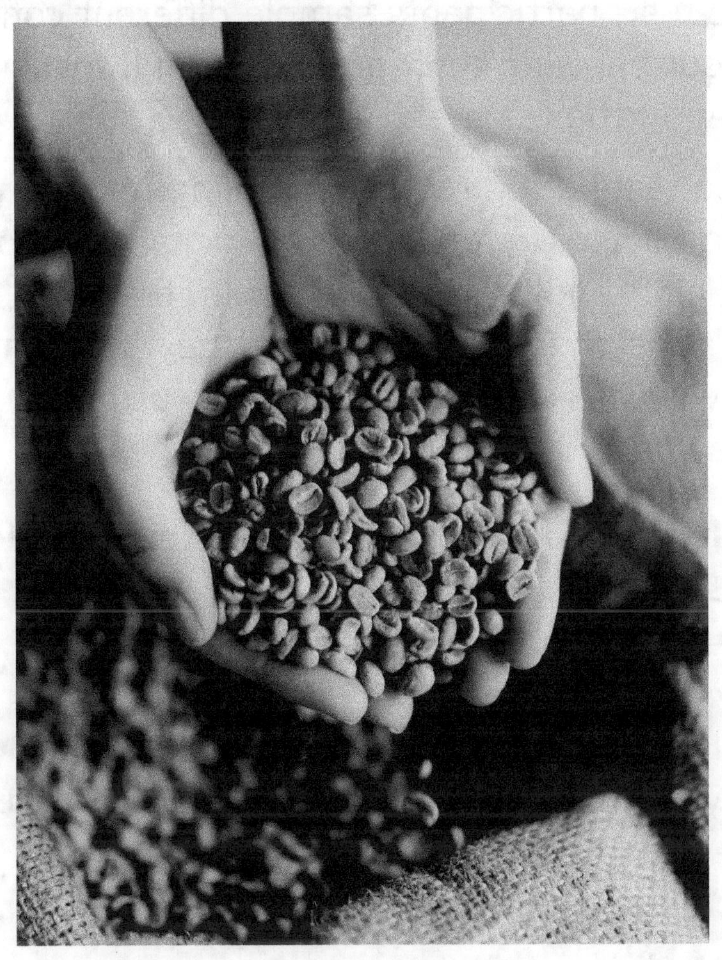

Chapter 9: Personal Preferences and Taste Tests

Conducting Blind Taste Tests

Blind taste tests are a valuable tool for evaluating coffee quality and determining personal preferences without bias. In a blind taste test, participants sample different coffees without knowing their price or brand, focusing solely on the taste and aroma.

These tests often reveal surprising results, with some people preferring less expensive options over high-end brands. Blind taste tests can help consumers discover what they truly enjoy and whether expensive coffee is worth the extra cost for them.

Analyzing Taste Preferences Across Price Ranges

Taste preferences vary widely among individuals, influenced by factors such as familiarity, exposure, and personal palate. Analyzing taste preferences across different price ranges can provide insights into what people value in their coffee.

Some common findings from taste tests include:

- Flavor Complexity: High-end coffees often have more complex and nuanced flavors, which can be appreciated by experienced coffee drinkers.

- Consistency: Expensive brands tend to offer more consistent quality, which can be a significant factor for those who prioritize reliability in their coffee.

- Acidity and Balance: Preferences for acidity and balance vary, with some consumers favoring the bright acidity of specialty coffees, while others prefer the robustness of cheaper blends.

Understanding these preferences helps consumers make informed choices about the value they place on different aspects of their coffee.

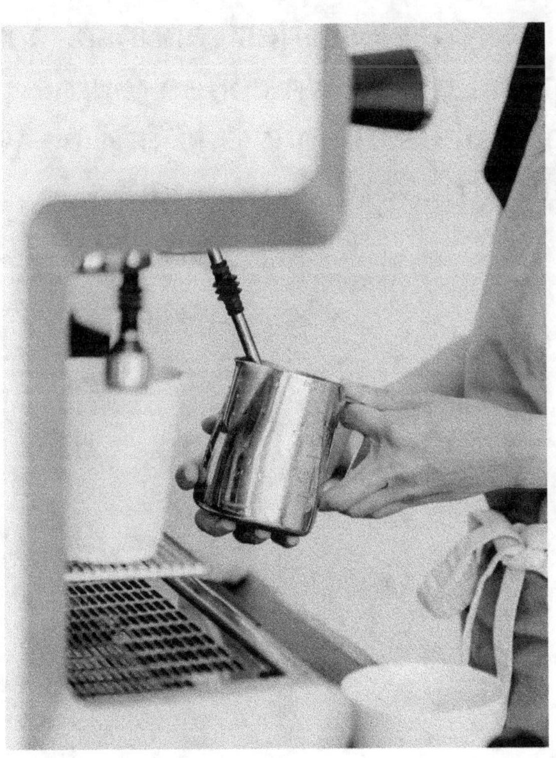

Stories and Testimonials from Coffee Enthusiasts

Hearing from coffee enthusiasts and professionals can provide valuable perspectives on the worth of expensive coffee. Many enthusiasts are passionate about the craft and enjoy exploring different beans, brewing methods, and flavors.

Testimonials from coffee lovers often highlight the joy and satisfaction derived from discovering a perfect cup of coffee, regardless of the price. These stories can inspire readers to embark on their own coffee journey, exploring various options and finding what brings them the most enjoyment.

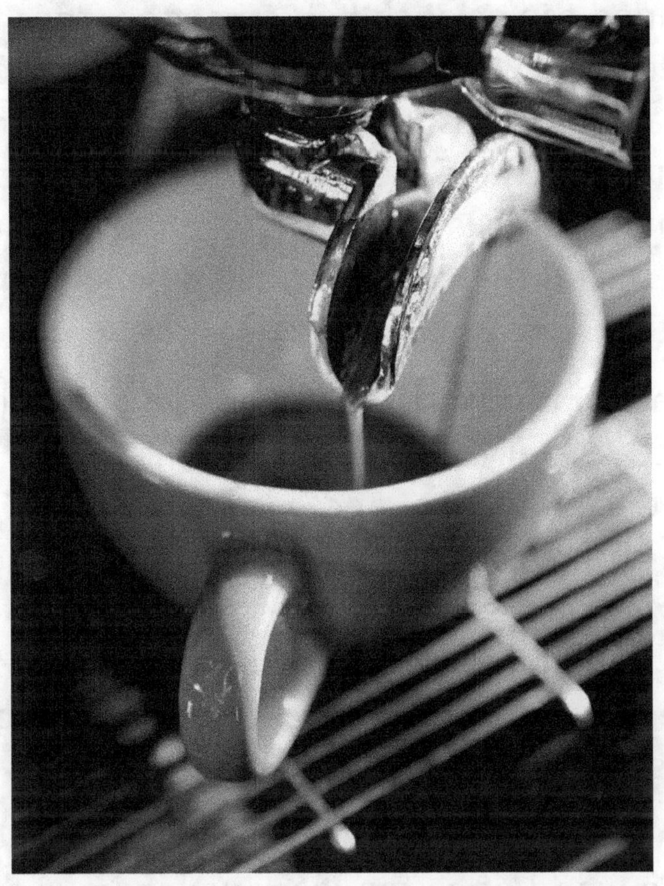

Conclusion

In our exploration of whether expensive coffee is actually worth it, we've delved into various aspects of the coffee world, from its cultural and economic significance to the intricate factors that influence pricing and quality. We've examined the science behind coffee, the impact of brewing methods, and the role of baristas and cafés in creating a premium coffee experience. We've also considered the health benefits and risks, the psychology of consumer choices, and the sustainability practices in the industry.

Ultimately, the worth of expensive coffee is subjective, varying based on individual preferences, values, and experiences. For some, the superior quality, ethical sourcing, and enhanced experience of premium coffee justify the higher price. For others, a well-brewed cup of affordable coffee can provide just as much satisfaction.

As readers, you're encouraged to explore the diverse world of coffee, conducting your own taste tests, visiting different cafés, and considering what aspects of the coffee experience matter most to you. Whether you prefer a budget-friendly brew or an artisanal cup from a high-end café, the important thing is to enjoy and appreciate the rich and varied journey that coffee offers.

References

- "The World Atlas of Coffee" by James Hoffmann

- "Coffee: A Comprehensive Guide to the Bean, the Beverage, and the Industry" by Robert W. Thurston

- Specialty Coffee Association (SCA) resources and publications

- Articles and studies from coffee industry experts and researchers

Recommended Reading List

Coffee Master - How to Become a Coffee Master at the Comfort of Your Home: "Unleash Your Inner Barista: A Guide to Mastering Coffee Brewing at Home"

https://www.amazon.com/dp/B0BV49Y634

Coffee Basics: Let's Brew Your First Cup of Joe - First Edition

https://www.amazon.com/dp/B0BR98641N

Coffee Making 101 How to brew a good cup of coffee Different ways of making coffee Energize your day with a cup of hug

https://www.amazon.com/dp/B0BQ524F8J

Brewing Brilliance: Mastering the World of Decaf Coffee: Celebrate Every Sip: Where Decaf Meets Brilliance!

https://www.amazon.com/dp/B0CSW3KXTM

Coffee Craft: Essential Drinks for Every Enthusiast: "Discover the Secrets of Coffee Craft and Brew Your Way to Bliss!"

https://www.amazon.com/dp/B0CV8CBFVN

Coffee Roasting Explained: A Comprehensive Guide for Beginners to Professionals: "Roast, Brew, Savor: Your Journey to Coffee Mastery Begins Here!"

https://www.amazon.com/dp/B0CVVLP3D1

Roasting Mastery: Techniques and Technologies for Perfect Coffee: "Elevate Your Coffee Experience with Precision Roasting Techniques!"

https://www.amazon.com/dp/B0CX98CFSD

Coffee Connoisseur's Companion: Navigating Ratios for Perfect Brews: Perfecting Your Pour: A Guide to Coffee Brewing Ratios

https://www.amazon.com/dp/B0D1CNNMXK

Coffee Craft: Essential Drinks for Every Enthusiast: "Discover the Secrets of Coffee

Craft and Brew Your Way to Bliss!" (Japanese Edition)

https://www.amazon.com/dp/B0CYPJMDQH

(French Version) Coffee Connoisseur's Companion: Navigating Ratios for Perfect Brews: Perfecting Your Pour: A Guide to Coffee Brewing Ratios

https://www.amazon.com/dp/B0D1LNSF4B

(Japanese Version) Coffee Connoisseur's Companion: Navigating Ratios for Perfect Brews: Perfecting Your Pour: A Guide to Coffee Brewing Ratios

https://www.amazon.com/dp/B0D264WXDW

Coffee Note:

Coffee Note:

Coffee Note:

Coffee Note:

Coffee Note:

Coffee Note:

Coffee Note:

Coffee Note: